Inflammatory diet for beginners (Calming the Fire Within)

Knowledge and Control of Inflammation by Diet

Marek Jane

Chapter One

Calming the Fire Within

Introduction

Many times referred to as the body's normal reaction to damage or infection, inflammation is essential to our health. But when inflammation becomes persistent and chronic, it can set off a series of detrimental consequences for our health that include autoimmune illnesses, diabetes, and cardiovascular problems. Among the complexity of contemporary living, knowing the complex link between nutrition and inflammation has become a key focus in preventive medicine.

Defining inflammation

The immune system of the body launches the intricate biological reaction known as inflammation in reaction to dangerous stimuli includes infections, injuries, or irritants. A number of physiological events, such as increased blood flow to the afflicted region, immune cell and signaling chemical release, and tissue repair mechanisms, are what define it. A defense mechanism, inflammation aids the body in removing toxic substances and starting the healing process. But chronic or dysregulated inflammation can fuel the onset of a number of illnesses and medical disorders.

Importance of understanding inflammation general health

Understanding inflammation is essential to general health because of its significant influence on physiological functions of the body and its part in the onset and progression of many disorders. This is a list of the primary arguments supporting the need of knowing inflammation to preserve good health:

1.   Disease   Prevention: Cardiovascular, diabetes, cancer, autoimmune, and neurological diseases like Alzheimer's disease are among the chronic illnesses for which chronic inflammation has been associated. Through knowledge of the elements that lead to inflammation, people can take preventative measures to lower their chance of getting certain diseases.

2. Immune Function: A basic element of the immune system's reaction is inflammation. It facilitates the removal of infections by bringing immune cells and signalling chemicals to the infection site. Protecting the body against infections and preventing over-inflammation that might harm healthy tissues need a balanced immune system.

3. The body's capacity to mend and regenerate injured tissues is greatly aided by inflammation. Inflammatory processes aid to clear up waste and damaged cells following an injury or infection, encourage the growth of new cells, and aid in tissue regeneration. Recovering from accidents and operations can be maximized by knowing how inflammation affects the healing process.

4. Chronic Disease Management: Handling symptoms and slowing down the course of chronic inflammatory diseases like psoriasis, inflammatory bowel disease, or rheumatoid arthritis requires an understanding of inflammation. Changing one's diet, controlling stress, and getting regular exercise are some lifestyle adjustments that can reduce inflammation and raise general quality of life.

5. Lifestyle Decisions: A number of lifestyle choices, such as food, exercise, stress levels, sleep quality, and exposure to environmental pollutants, can affect the body's inflammatory condition. Knowing how these things impact inflammation will enable people to make decisions that will benefit their general health and wellbeing. The balanced diet high in whole foods, frequent exercise, stress-reduction strategies, and enough sleep that make up an anti-inflammatory lifestyle can assist to reduce inflammation and promote long-term health.

The function of diet in Inflammation

Diet plays a major part in inflammation since the body's inflammatory processes can be fueled or slowed down by certain food choices.

1. Pro-Inflammatory Foods: It's well known that some foods increase inflammation in the body. Those consist of:

• **Processed Foods:** Inflammatory foods include those heavy in additives, trans and saturated fats, and processed carbohydrates.

• **Refined Carbohydrates:** Blood sugar swings from white bread, pastries, and sugary drinks can exacerbate inflammation.

• **Red Meat**: Eating a lot of red meat—especially processed red meats like sausage and bacon—

has been linked to increased inflammation.

• **Fried Foods:** Unhealthy oils used to fry foods include toxic chemicals that can exacerbate inflammation.

2. Contrarily, some foods offer **anti-inflammatory** qualities that can lessen inflammation in the body. Those consist of:

• **Fruits and Vegetables:** High in vitamins, minerals, antioxidants, and phytochemicals, fruits and vegetables boost general health and fight inflammation.

- **Fatty Fish:** High in omega-3 fatty acids, which have strong anti-inflammatory properties, cold-water fatty fish include salmon, mackerel, and sardines.

- **Whole Grains:** Packed with fiber and minerals that may lower inflammation are whole grains like quinoa, brown rice, and oats.

- **Nuts and Seeds:** Excellent suppliers of antioxidants that can fight inflammation, fiber, and healthy fats are almonds, walnuts, flaxseeds, and chia seeds.

Strong anti-inflammatory herbs and spices include turmeric, ginger, garlic, and cinnamon.

3. Gut Health: Controlling inflammation in the body is mostly dependent on the gut flora. A diet heavy in fiber from fruits, vegetables, and whole grains promotes a healthy gut flora, which lowers inflammation. Additionally promoting gut health and perhaps having anti-inflammatory properties are fermented foods including yogurt, kefir, sauerkraut, and kimchi.

4. Weight Control: Chronic low-grade inflammation linked to obesity advances a number of diseases. Eating a well-balanced diet and keeping a healthy weight can assist to lessen inflammation and the chance of diseases linked to obesity.

5. Individual Variability: It's critical to understand that every person's inflammatory reaction to diet is different. The way the body reacts to certain foods is influenced by factors like heredity, underlying medical disorders, and general eating habits.

Chapter Two

Types of Inflammatory (acute vs. chronic)

Acute inflammation and chronic inflammation are the two basic categories into which inflammation can be generally separated.

1. Prolonged Inflammation:

• **Nature:** Inflammation that occurs quickly and briefly in reaction to damaging stimuli such tissue damage, infection, or injury.

• **Duration:** Depending on how severe the trigger was and how the body responded, it usually lasts a few hours to many days.

Symptoms of acute inflammation include redness, swelling, heat, discomfort, and loss of function in the afflicted area.

• **Objective:** Removing the cause of the damage or infection and starting the healing process are the main objectives of acute inflammation. Immunological cells are activated, inflammatory mediators are released, and immune cells are drawn to the area of damage.

• **Examples:** Acute inflammation follows cuts, burns, infections (viral, bacterial), and acute diseases like bronchitis or appendicitis.

2. Chronic Inflammation

- **Nature:** Weeks, months, or even years might pass while an inflammatory response is ongoing and sustained.

- **Duration:** Chronic inflammation can last long even in the lack of a clear trigger, unlike acute inflammation, which goes away as the triggering event is eliminated.

- **Symptoms:** The hallmarks of acute inflammation may not be present in chronic inflammation and it may be less noticeable. Rather, it can appear subtly as joint pain, exhaustion, a low-grade fever that never goes away, and general malaise.

- **Effects:** Cardiovascular diseases, diabetes, autoimmune diseases, neurological disorders, and some malignancies are among the chronic illnesses whose onset and progression are linked to chronic inflammation.

- **Causes:** Prolonged contact to irritants like environmental pollutants, poor diet, ongoing infections, obesity, stress, and autoimmune responses can lead to chronic inflammation.

Examples of chronic inflammatory disorders are atherosclerosis, asthma, psoriasis, inflammatory bowel disease (such as ulcerative colitis and Crohn's disease), and rheumatoid arthritis.

Causes of inflammation (aspects of lifestyle, stress, and food)

Numerous things, including stress, nutrition, and lifestyle choices, can set off inflammation. These are some of the main reasons of inflammation broken down:

1. Diet

•	**Pro-inflammatory meals:** Eating processed meals heavy in refined sugars, trans and saturated fats, and additives can increase inflammation in the body.

•	**Refined Carbohydrates:** Foods like processed snacks, sugary drinks, pastries, and white bread can raise blood sugar levels and hence raise inflammation.

• **Red Meat and Processed Meats:** Higher levels of inflammation have been linked with large amounts of red meat, especially processed meats like bacon and sausage.

- **Unhealthy Cooking Methods:** Unhealthy oils used in frying or high-temperature cooking of foods might result in toxic substances that aggravate inflammation.

- **Inadequate Consumption of Anti-inflammatory Nutrients:** Inflammation can also result from an inadequate consumption of anti-inflammatory nutrients including omega-3 fatty acids, antioxidants, vitamins, and minerals found in fruits, vegetables, fatty fish, nuts and seeds.

2. Stress

- **Psychological Stress:** The body can eventually become more inflammatory when chronic stress releases stress chemicals like cortisol.

- **Inflammatory Response:** Pro-inflammatory cytokines and the stimulation of the sympathetic nervous system are two ways that the body reacts to stress and add to systemic inflammation.

- **Behavioral Responses:** Stress can also result in unhealthful coping strategies such overeating, eating poorly, getting enough sleep, and being inactive, all of which can make inflammation worse.

3. Life Style Aspects:

- **Physical Inactivity:** Sedentary lifestyle and infrequent exercise are linked to higher inflammation and a greater chance of chronic illnesses.

- **Smoking:** The lungs might become inflamed and subjected to oxidative stress when one smokes cigarettes.

- **Alcoholism:** Drinking too much alcohol can harm the liver, increase inflammation, and upset gut health.

• **Sleep deprivation:** Poor or no sleep might impair immune system and raise inflammation.

• Environmental Toxins: The body can mount inflammatory reactions in response to exposure to chemicals, toxins, and pollution.

4. Chronic Diseases and Autoimmune Responses:

• **Chronic Infections:** An inflammatory reaction in the body can be sustained by chronic infections brought on by bacteria, viruses, or other pathogens.

• **Autoimmune Disorders:** Chronic inflammation can result

from diseases including rheumatoid arthritis, lupus, and inflammatory bowel disease, in which the immune system inadvertently targets healthy tissues.

Health effects of chronic inflammation (association with several disorders)

Wide-ranging health consequences can result from chronic inflammation, which helps to initiate and advance a number of diseases affecting several organ systems.

1. Diseases of the Cardiovascular System

The accumulation of plaque in the arteries known as atherosclerosis is mostly caused by chronic inflammation.

• The arteries narrow, plaque development occurs, and the risk of heart attack and stroke is raised by inflammatory processes within the artery walls.

• The instability of atherosclerotic plaques is another way that chronic inflammation raises the possibility of rupture and thrombosis.

2. Metabolic Illnesses

The characteristic of type 2 diabetes, insulin resistance, is intimately associated with chronic inflammation.

• Because inflammation disrupts the pathways that activate insulin, blood sugar levels rise and the risk of diabetes rises.

• Chronic low-grade inflammation linked to obesity aggravates metabolic dysfunction and insulin resistance even further.

3. Disorders of the Autoimmune System

• Chronic inflammation and dysregulation of immune responses are hallmarks of autoimmune disorders like rheumatoid arthritis, systemic lupus erythematosus (SLE), and inflammatory bowel illnesses (Crohn's disease and ulcerative colitis).

• When the immune system incorrectly targets healthy tissues, inflammation and tissue damage in many organs and systems result.

4. Neurological Illnesses:

• The development of neurodegenerative disorders like multiple sclerosis, Parkinson's disease, and Alzheimer's disease has been linked to chronic inflammation.

Neuronal loss, synaptic malfunction, and cognitive impairment can all result from brain inflammation.

In such circumstances, neuroinflammation and neuronal damage are exacerbated by the activation of microglia, the immune cells of the central nervous system.

5. Cancer

• Cancer starts, progresses, and spreads more easily in a pro-tumorigenic milieu that chronic inflammation produces.

• Immune system-produced inflammatory cytokines and

chemokines promote tissue remodeling, angiogenesis, and cell proliferation, therefore promoting tumor growth.

• Chronic hepatitis and inflammatory bowel disease, for example, raise the risk of colorectal and hepatocellular carcinomas among other malignancies.

6. Diseases of the Respiratory System

• Respiratory diseases including bronchitis, chronic obstructive pulmonary disease (COPD), and asthma are thought to have a pathogenic component of chronic inflammation.

- Bronchoconstriction, airway remodeling, and mucus hypersecretion brought on by airway inflammation add to respiratory symptoms and airflow restriction.

7. Skin disorder:

- Psoriasis, eczema, and acne are among the skin disorders whose pathophysiology includes chronic inflammation.

- Skin inflammation, keratinocyte proliferation, and abnormal immunological responses are all exacerbated by inflammatory mediators.

Chapter Three

Foods that make up an inflammatory diet

1. Highly Processed Meals:

• Refined sugars, bad fats, and additives—all of which can cause inflammation—are common in processed foods.

• Examples include processed meats, fast food, desserts, sugary drinks, and packaged snacks made with artificial components.

2. Clean Carbohydrates:

• High glycmic index refined carbohydrates include white bread, white rice, pasta, and sugary cereals, which cause blood sugar increases quickly and increase inflammation.

• These foods don't have the fiber and other vital nutrients which are anti-inflammatory found in whole grains.

3. Not Good Fats:

• Inflammation may be induced by trans fats and by overindulging in saturated fats from baked goods, processed snacks, fried foods, and fatty cuts of meat.

• By upsetting cellular membranes and adding to oxidative stress, these fats raise the level of pro-inflammatory compounds produced.

4. Overindulging in omega-6 fatty acids

Omega-6 fatty acids are necessary fats present in vegetable oils including sunflower, corn, and soybean oils.

• Although a sufficient intake of omega-6 fatty acids is essential for health, an imbalance that encourages inflammation might result from an excessive consumption.

Chronic inflammation may be exacerbated by a diet heavy in

processed foods and omega-6 fatty acid-rich cooking oils.

5. Lots Much Sugar Consumption

• Consuming too much of the added sugars in processed meals, candies, desserts, and sugary drinks can aggravate inflammation.

• Inflammatory cytokines are produced more readily by high sugar intake, which also increases insulin resistance and oxidative stress.

6. Inorganic Preservatives and Additives

• In sensitive people, artificial additives, preservatives, and food colorings in processed foods might cause inflammatory reactions.

• These additions might impair immune system and gut health, which would exacerbate chronic inflammation.

7. Alcohol

• Overindulging in alcohol can alter the flora of the stomach, increase intestinal permeability, and raise systemic inflammation.

• Abuse of alcohol over time is linked to oxidative stress, inflammation of the liver, and a higher incidence of disorders linked to inflammation.

8. Food Allergies and Sensitivities

• Some people may be allergic to or sensitive to particular foods that can cause inflammation, such dairy, gluten, soy, or nightshade vegetables.

• In some people, identifying and avoiding trigger foods can help lower inflammation and relieve symptoms.

Meals high in inflammation (trans fats, processed meals, sugar, etc.)

I. Sugary food and Drinks:

• Inflammation can result from foods heavy in added sugars, including sodas, energy drinks, sweet cereals, pastries, sweets, and sweetened snacks.

• Overindulging in sugar raises blood sugar, encourages insulin resistance, and sets off inflammatory reactions in the body.

2. Products of Processing:

• A lot of times, processed foods are heavy in chemicals, bad fats, and refined carbohydrates—all of which can exacerbate inflammation.

• Fast food, processed meats (such as bacon and sausages), sugary cereals, and packaged snacks are a few examples.

3. Unsaturated Fats

• Partially hydrogenated oils used in many processed and fried meals include artificial fats known as trans fats.

• French fries, fried chicken, baked goods (pastries, cakes, cookies), margarine, and processed snacks (chips, crackers) are among the items heavy in trans fats.

• LDL cholesterol levels are raised by trans fats, which also increase the risk of heart disease and other inflammatory diseases.

4. Clean Carbohydrates:

• High glycemic index refined carbohydrates include white bread, white rice, pasta made from refined wheat, and sugary cereals.

• Over time, the quick jumps in blood sugar levels brought on by these foods can result in inflammation and insulin resistance.

5. Bad Cooking Oils:

• When used in excess, several cooking oils heavy in omega-6 fatty acids—such soybean, corn, sunflower, and vegetable oils—can exacerbate inflammation.

• Fried, processed, and restaurant cuisine all frequently use these oils.

6. Highly Processed Meats:

• A number of processed meats, including bacon, sausage, hot dogs, deli meats, and some lunch meats, include harmful fats, preservatives, and additives that can exacerbate inflammation.

• High salt and nitrate contents in these meats may also raise the risk of cardiovascular disease and inflammation.

7. Alcohol

• Drinking too much alcohol could change the flora of the gut, make the intestines more permeable, and raise inflammation in the body.

• Abuse of alcohol over time is linked to oxidative stress, inflammation of the liver, and a higher incidence of disorders linked to inflammation.

Chapter Four

Anti-inflammatory foods (fruits, veggies, fatty fish, etc.)

1. Fruits:

• Berries: High in antioxidants such anthocyanins, which lower inflammation, include blueberries, strawberries, raspberries, and blackberries.

• Cherries: Rich in antioxidants including anthocyanins that reduce inflammation.

• Citrus fruits (grapefruits, lemons, oranges): Rich in vitamin C, a potent anti-inflammatory.

Pineapple: Has the anti-inflammatory enzyme bromelain.

• Apples: Packed with anti-inflammatory flavonoids and fiber.

2. Vegetables:

Rich in antioxidants, vitamins (such as vitamin K), and minerals that lower inflammation include leafy greens (spinach, kale, Swiss chard).

• Broccoli, Brussels sprouts, cauliflower and other cruciferous vegetables: These have the anti-inflammatory molecule sulforaphane.

• High in the potent antioxidant lycopene, tomatoes lower inflammation.

Rich in vitamin C and other antioxidants that fight inflammation are bell peppers.

• Sweet potatoes: Loaded with anti-inflammatory antioxidants like beta-carotene.

3. Fish high in fat

Omega-3 fatty acids abound in salmon, mackerel, sardines, trout, and other fatty fish, especially EPA (eicosapentaenoic acid) and DHA (docosahexaenoic acid).

- Strong anti-inflammatory qualities of omega-3 fatty acids aid to lower inflammation all over the body.

4. Seeds & Nuts

- Excellent suppliers of antioxidants, fiber, and healthy fats are almonds, walnuts, flaxseeds, chia seeds, and hemp seeds.

- High in the anti-inflammatory fatty acid omega-3.

- Other minerals that lower inflammation include magnesium and those found in nuts and seeds.

5. All Whole Grains:

• High in fibre, vitamins, minerals and antioxidants are whole grains such as oats, brown rice, quinoa, barley and bulgur.

• Foods high in fiber lower inflammation and support intestinal health.

• The lower glycemic index of whole grains over processed grains also helps to lessen inflammation and stabilize blood sugar levels.

6. Spices and herbs

• Turmeric: It includes curcumin, an antioxidant and strong anti-inflammatory.

- Ginger: Has anti-inflammatory bioactive molecule gingerol.

- Rich in sulfur compounds with anti-inflammatory and immune-boosting effects is garlic.

- Cinnamon: Contains antioxidants that help reduce inflammation and increase insulin sensitivity.

7. Nutrient with Dense Fats

Avocados: Packed full of antioxidants and monounsaturated fats that lower inflammation.

- Extra virgin olive oil: Has anti-inflammatory-effecting antioxidants like oleocanthal.

• Coconut oil: It includes the anti-inflammatory substances lauric acid and medium-chain triglycerides (MCTs).

Inflammation and the gut: a role for food

The complexity and reciprocity of the link between gut health and inflammation make the gut essential for controlling inflammation throughout the body. The following summarizes the relationship between inflammation and gut health and the dietary measures that can support gut health and lower inflammation:

1. Internal Barrier Action:

- Water, nutrients, and other materials are regulated by the gut lining's function as a barrier from the intestines into the blood.

- Systemic inflammation is less likely when a good gut barrier keeps poisons, bacteria, and undigested food particles out of the bloodstream.

Increased intestinal permeability, sometimes referred to as "leaky gut," is a condition in which bacteria and other antigens translocate from the gut into the bloodstream, therefore initiating inflammatory reactions.

2. Intestinal Microbiology:

• The billions of bacteria that make up the gut microbiota are essential to preserving gut health and controlling immune system activity.

• The development of helpful bacteria that generate anti-inflammatory substances is encouraged and the expansion of harmful bacteria is prevented by a balanced and diverse gut flora.

• Inflammatory bowel diseases (IBD), metabolic problems, and other inflammatory diseases are linked to dysbiosis, an imbalance in the composition of the gut microbiota.

3. The modulation of the immune system

• A major component of immune cell production and immunological activity are housed in the gut-associated lymphoid tissue (GALT).

• Through interactions with the immune system, the gut microbiota maintains immunological tolerance to innocuous substances and trains immune cells.

• Inflammation that persists over time and autoimmune responses against the gut microbiota or self-tissues might result from dysregulation of the immune system.

4. Nutritional Therapies for Inflammation and Gut Health

• **Foods High in Fiber:** By supporting good gut bacteria and encouraging regular bowel movements, dietary fiber found in fruits, vegetables, whole grains, legumes, and nuts supports gut health. Short-chain fatty acids (SCFAs), including butyrate, that gut bacteria ferment generate have anti-inflammatory properties.

• **Probiotic Foods:** Good bacteria found in fermented foods like kombucha, sauerkraut, kimchi, and yogurt can help heal the gut microbiota and lower inflammation.

- **Foods High in Prebiotics:** These fibers are not digested and provide sustenance for helpful gut flora. Products high in prebiotics include whole grains, garlic, onions, leeks, asparagus, and bananas.

- **Anti-Inflammatory Foods:** Including foods high in omega-3 fatty acids, antioxidants, and phytonutrients into the diet will help lower inflammation and promote gut health. Examples are green tea, berries, leafy greens, turmeric, ginger, and fatty salmon.

- **eliminating Inflammatory Triggers:** Improving general health and reducing gut inflammation can be accomplished by limiting or eliminating foods that increase inflammation, like processed foods, refined carbohydrates, unhealthy fats, and artificial additives.

Chapter Five

Guides for dietary reduction of inflammation

1. Emphasize Natural, Whole Foods:

• Center your meals on minimally processed, whole foods including fruits, vegetables, whole grains, legumes, nuts, seeds, and lean proteins.

• Select whole foods high in fiber, vitamins, antioxidants, and phytonutrients, which improve general health and fight inflammation.

2. Boost Consumption of Foods Low in Inflammation

- Eat a wide variety of anti-inflammatory foods, including leafy greens, berries, nuts, seeds, olive oil, turmeric, ginger, garlic, and green tea; also include fatty fish (such as salmon, mackerel, and sardines).

- Omega-3 fatty acids, antioxidants, and other bioactive substances found in plenty in these foods aid to lower inflammation.

3. Reduce Consumption of Foods That Inflame

- Eat less of processed meals, refined carbs, sugary snacks and drinks, trans fats, and fried foods—items that increase inflammation.

• Eat less of processed and red meats, dairy items high in fat, and foods with artificial preservatives and additives.

4. Select Nutrient-Dense Fats

• Select sources of extra virgin olive oil, nuts, seeds, avocados, and fatty fish.

• These fats include anti-inflammatory omega-3 fatty acids as well as other mono- and polyunsaturated fats.

5. Add Foods High in Fiber

• Eat a range of foods high in fibre, such as fruits, vegetables, whole grains, legumes, nuts and seeds.

By supporting good gut bacteria and encouraging the synthesis of short-chain fatty acids, fiber improves gut health, controls blood sugar levels, and lowers inflammation.

6. Eat Foods High in Prebiotic and Probiotics

• Eat foods high in probiotics, such yogurt, kefir, sauerkraut, kimchi, kombucha, and other fermented items.

• Eat foods high in prebiotics, such as garlic, onions, leeks, asparagus, bananas, oats, and

Jerusalem artichokes, which nourish helpful gut bacteria.

8. Drink Plenty of Water to Rehydrate

• Stay hydrated all day long by sipping lots of water.

• Cut back on alcohol and sugary drinks, which can exacerbate dehydration and inflammation.

Planning meals and selection of recipes

Without a doubt. The following meal planning and cooking ideas emphasize anti-inflammatory foods:

Planning a Meal:

1. Plan Balanced Meals: Try to include a range of foods high in nutrients—fruits, vegetables, whole grains, lean meats, and good fats into each meal.

2. Add Anti-Inflammatory Ingredients: Select foods like fatty fish, leafy greens, berries, nuts and seeds, olive oil, turmeric, and ginger that are well-known for their anti-inflammatory qualities.

3. Think about batch cooking a lot of basic items at the start of the week to use in several meals, such as whole grains, beans, and roasted veggies.

4. Variety: To guarantee a wide spectrum of tastes and nutrients, alternate between several kinds of grains, vegetables, and meats during the week.

5. Portion Control: To prevent overindulging and guarantee balanced meals, be aware of portion sizes.

Recipes Idea:

1. A bowl of salmon quinoa:

Fish fillets grilled or baked over cooked quinoa.

• Topped with roasted veggies (bell peppers, broccoli, and cauliflower) and sautéed leafy greens (spinach, kale, Swiss chard).

• Drizzled with a herb-garlic-tahini dressing prepared from olive oil, lemon juice, tahini, and garlic.

2. Chickpea Salad with Mediterranean Flavors

• A cool salad made with red onions, cucumber, cherry tomatoes, red peppers, Kalamata olives, and fresh mint and parsley.

• Tossed with crumbled feta cheese and lemon-olive oil vinaigrette.

Serve with whole grain pita bread or over a bed of mixed greens.

3. Stir-Fry Vegetables with Tofu

• In sesame oil, stir-fry a rainbow of bright vegetables including bell peppers, broccoli, snap peas, carrots, and mushrooms.

For protein derived from plants, add cubed tofu.

• Season with garlic, ginger, soy sauce (or, if gluten-free, tamari), and a little rice vinegar.

• Top brown rice or quinoa with chopped green onions and sesame seeds.

4. With grilled chicken, a berry spinach salad

• Mix cut raspberries, blueberries, and strawberries with fresh spinach leaves.

• For protein, top with slices of grilled chicken breast or tofu.

• Chop walnuts and crumbled goat or feta cheese for a garnish.

• Drizzle with a balsamic vinaigrette prepared with honey (or maple syrup for vegan option), Dijon mustard, and olive oil.

5. Coconut Lentil Soup with Turmeric

- In coconut oil, sauté onions, garlic, ginger and turmeric till aromatic.

- Stir in coconut milk, chopped veggies (bell peppers, celery, and carrots), red lentils and vegetable broth.

- Simmer till lentils are soft and flavors have blended.

- Squeeze in some lemon juice and season with pepper and salt to add flavor.

- Top with a dollop of Greek yogurt or, for a vegan option, coconut yogurt and fresh cilantro.

Specific medical illnesses (such as autoimmune diseases, cardiovascular disease, and arthritis) and inflammation

Autoimmune diseases, cardiovascular disease, and arthritis are only a few of the medical problems whose origin and course are greatly influenced by inflammation. The following describes how several medical disorders are related to inflammation:

I. **Arthritis**

• An inflammatory joint disease family including arthritis is typified by pain, stiffness, swelling, and reduced range of motion.

• Inflammatory arthritis, which causes joint damage and deformity, includes persistent inflammation in the synovium, the lining of the joints, as in rheumatoid arthritis (RA) and psoriatic arthritis.

• When the immune system incorrectly targets the synovium in RA, inflammation and bone and cartilage degradation result.

• Pain, swelling, and continuing joint deterioration brought on by chronic inflammation in the joints can result in disability and a lower quality of life.

2. Cardiovascular disease, or CVD:

• Atherosclerosis, myocardial infarction (heart attack), and stroke are among the cardiovascular disorders whose genesis and progression are mostly influenced by chronic inflammation.

• Plaque, which is made up of cholesterol, immune cells, and cellular debris, builds up in the artery walls of atherosclerosis, narrowing and hardening the arteries.

• The development, instability, and rupture of plaques by inflammatory processes within the artery walls result in thrombosis and cardiovascular events.

• Higher inflammatory marker levels like CRP and IL 6 are linked to a higher risk of CVD and unfavorable cardiovascular outcomes.

3. Disorders of the Autoimmune System

• When the immune system unintentionally targets healthy tissues, persistent inflammation and tissue damage result, causing autoimmune disorders.

Among the autoimmune diseases include rheumatoid arthritis, type

1 diabetes, multiple sclerosis (MS), systemic lupus erythematosus (SLE), and inflammatory bowel disease (IBD).

• When autoimmune disorders strike certain tissues or organs, inflammation, tissue damage, and malfunction result.

• The emergence of autoimmune diseases can be facilitated by genetic predisposition, environmental triggers, dysregulation of immune responses, and changes in gut flora.

4. Inflammatory bowel disease or IBD:

The hallmark of IBD, which includes ulcerative colitis and Crohn's disease, is persistent gastrointestinal inflammation.

• Deep layers of tissue may become involved in Crohn's disease inflammation, which can happen anywhere throughout the digestive tract, from the mouth to the anus.

• Ulcerative colitis mostly damages the colon and rectum, inflaming and rupturing the colon's lining.

IBD-related chronic inflammation causes symptoms like weight loss, diarrhea, rectal bleeding, and stomach pain.

5. Psoriasis

• Red, scaly patches on the skin are a hallmark of psoriasis, a chronic inflammatory skin condition.

• In psoriasis, thicker, inflamed plaques are formed when immune cells release inflammatory cytokines that encourage the quick turnover of skin cells.

• Chronic inflammation in psoriatic lesions can go beyond the skin, escalating the risk of cardiovascular disease and other comorbidities and adding to systemic inflammation.

Chapter Six

Nutritional factors to be taken into account when controlling inflammation in various groups (sportsmen, children, elderly, etc.).

Indeed, certain dietary factors should be taken into account while controlling inflammation in various populations:

The kids:

• Stress Whole Foods: Promote a diet heavy in minimally processed, whole foods including fruits and vegetables.

lean proteins, good fats, and entire carbohydrates.

• Cut Back on Sugary Foods and Drinks: Eating too much sugar can increase inflammation and exacerbate chronic health issues. Reduce sugary snacks, desserts and drinks.

• Include Omega-3 Fatty Acids: To help lower inflammation and promote brain development, include sources of omega-3 fatty acids in their diet, including fatty fish (salmon, mackerel, sardines), flaxseeds, chia seeds, and walnuts.

• Support Gut Health: To help maintain gut health and control inflammation, include foods high in fiber, such as fruits, vegetables, and whole grains. To preserve a good balance of the gut flora, promote the eating of foods high in probiotics, such as yogurt, kefir, and fermented vegetables.

2. Elderly People

• Give Nutrient-Dense Foods Top Priority: Give foods high in vitamins, minerals, and antioxidants that help immune system and general health priority.

• Make Sure You Get Enough Protein: To help with muscle building, strength, and recovery, include sources of high-quality protein include lean meats, poultry, fish, eggs, dairy, legumes, and tofu.

• Eat Anti-Inflammatory Foods: To lower inflammation and control age-related chronic illnesses, include in their diet foods like fatty fish, leafy greens, berries, nuts, seeds, olive oil, turmeric, and ginger.

• Keep Hydrated: Drink enough of water all day long to promote proper hydration, as dehydration can worsen inflammation and raise the chance of problems.

3. Athletes:

• Maximise Macronutrient Balance: To promote energy

generation, muscle repair and recovery, make sure you are getting enough of protein, carbs and healthy fats.

• Fuel with entire Foods: Give entire, nutrient-dense foods fruits, vegetables, whole grains, lean meats, and healthy fats priority in order to supply the necessary nutrients and antioxidants for recovery and best performance.

• Control Inflammation: To assist lower inflammation brought on by exercise and aid in recovery, include sources of omega-3 fatty acids in their diet, like fatty fish, flaxseeds, chia seeds, and walnuts.

• Hydrate Right: To support performance and lower the chance of inflammation and muscular cramping brought on by dehydration; drink enough of water before, during, and after exercise.

• Think About Meal Timing and Composition: During training and recovery times, optimize fuel use and nutrient delivery by paying attention to the timing and composition of meals and snacks.

4. Pregnant or Nursing women

• Emphasize Nutrient-Rich Foods: To supply vital nutrients for the health of the mother and fetus, stress a balanced diet high in fruits, vegetables, whole grains, lean proteins, and healthy fats.

• Make Sure You're Getting Enough Omega-3s: To help fetal brain and eye development and lower inflammation, include sources of omega-3 fatty acids like fatty fish (such as salmon and trout), flaxseeds, chia seeds, and walnuts.

• Steer Clear of Excess Sugars and Processed Foods: Eat as little processed foods, sweets, and snacks as possible as they can raise inflammation and raise the chance of gestational diabetes and other problems.

• Stay Hydrated: Throughout pregnancy and nursing, drink enough of water to promote appropriate hydration and lower the chance of inflammation and problems brought on by dehydration.

5. Those with long-term medical conditions (such as diabetes, cardiovascular disease, and autoimmune diseases):

• Eat a Balanced Diet: To support general health and supply vital nutrients, eat a range of foods high in nutrients from all food groups.

• Control Carbohydrate Intake: To help those with diabetes or insulin resistance lower inflammation and stabilize blood sugar levels, watch how much you eat and select complex carbs with a low glycemic index.

• Cut Back on Sodium and Processed Foods: Eating too much of either can increase inflammation and make diseases like hypertension and cardiovascular disease worse.

• Customize Dietary Recommendations: Based on particular health issues, medical history, and nutritional requirements, customize dietary recommendations working with a certified dietitian or healthcare provider.

The need of sleep, stress management, and exercise in lowering inflammation

I. Exercise

• The body has been demonstrated to have anti-inflammatory effects from regular exercise.

• Exercise reduces inflammation generally by raising anti-inflammatory cytokines and lowering pro-inflammatory cytokines.

• Exercises for flexibility, resistance, and aerobics all help to lower inflammation and enhance immune system function.

• Because extra body fat can exacerbate inflammation, exercise also helps with weight management.

2. Stress Reduction

• The body's stress response system is activated by chronic stress, which releases stress hormones like adrenaline and cortisol and can so exacerbate inflammation.

• Prolonged low-grade inflammation can result from immune system dysregulation brought on by prolonged stress.

• Yoga, deep breathing exercises, mindfulness meditation, and progressive muscular relaxation are among stress-reduction strategies.

• Stress can also be reduced and emotional well-being promoted, which in turn helps lower inflammation, by participating in fun activities, spending time in nature, and building social relationships.

3. At night:

• The body needs enough sleep to manage immunity, heal and rebuild tissues, and preserve general health.

• Poor quality or chronic sleep loss can impair immune system and raise inflammation.

• To assist control inflammation, the body creates anti-inflammatory cytokines and lowers pro-inflammatory cytokines when it sleeps.

• Try to get between seven and nine hours of good sleep every night, and create a peaceful bedtime routine, a regular sleep schedule, and an ideal sleeping environment.